Ketogenic Diet

By

Tina K. Bing

Table of Contents

Introduction

Eating fat can make us lose weight!?

The drastic diets are over! Some foods are composed of "good fats" so bet on a rich and healthy diet to finally get our dream silhouette.

Exit carbohydrates! With the ketogenic diet, you fill up with fat to lose weight. Focus on this diet of a new kind.

Definition

Ketogenic diet or keto diet, as it is called, mainly consists of proteins and fats, but there are practically no carbohydrates in it. Due to such nutrition, the organism falls into a state of ketosis, in which the replacement of the necessary energy costs occurs at the expense of accumulated subcutaneous fat without the disintegration of the muscle. When the fats are split, ketones are formed, which give the energy necessary for the body. And this is its plus. Another reason for losing weight is a large amount of protein consumed, which reduces appetite.

Surprisingly, Keto diet fans do not even count the number of calories and eat quite freely. It is known that on a ketogenic diet participants lost 2.2 times more weight than those who counted calories and limited the content of fats.

More than 20 studies, according to Authority Nutrition, have proven the benefit of a ketogenic diet for weight loss and health. It is used for diabetes, epilepsy, Alzheimer's disease, liver obesity, certain cancers. Types of ketogenic diets

There are several variants of a ketogenic diet, for example:

Standard ketogenic diet:

It implies a low carbohydrate content (5%), a moderate protein content (20%) and a high-fat content (75%).

Cyclic ketogenic diet:

This kind includes periods of carbohydrate loading.

For example, five days of ketogenic diet and two days of a usual day.

Targeted ketogenic diet:

Allows you to add carbohydrates during training days.

High-protein ketogenic diet:

Includes a large number of proteins. The ratio of macronutrients: 60% of fats, 35% of proteins and 5% of carbohydrates.

How does a ketogenic diet help to lose weight?

The menu, compiled on the basis of the keto diet, triggers natural mechanisms in the body that actively break down subcutaneous fat. This process begins to run already on the 2nd - 3rd day after a properly formulated power supply. Adoption of the body to replace glucose with ketone bodies takes several days. It is recommended at the first time to eat more vegetables and water. Vegetables, their permissible norm should not exceed 40-50 g, at one time. It is allowed to eat lettuce leaves in larger quantities. Take a dietary supplement or add high omega-3 whole foods, such as flax nuts, macadamia, as well as vitamin E and magnesium. An additional advantage of this diet is that while eating a person does not overeat and during the day, he is not tormented by a strong sense of hunger. This is because the diet does not allow the insulin level to rise very much. It is known that insulin is responsible for feeling hungry.

Keto diet is unique in that after a person stops, adhere to the established scheme of nutrition; extra pounds are not returned. This is because during the diet, a person does not starve, but the body simply gets used to the permissible norm of consumed food.

There are several reasons why a ketogenic diet works so well. One of them is an increased intake of protein, which restrains the appetite.

Also, lowering blood sugar levels improves insulin sensitivity.

Principles of the Ketogenic Diet

To achieve the objectives of the ketogenic diet, it is imperative to follow some rules. Among the most important, there are for example the meals to be taken throughout the diet. To have a more precise idea on the subject, it is important to know which foods are to be consumed or not.

The ketogenic diet proscribed the consumption of certain foods. In general, these are those containing far too much carbohydrate. The most important are:

SUGAR: This concerns; for example, white sugar, brown sugar, honey and maple syrup, which is entirely prohibited during the entire ketogenic diet. Foods that contain them are also to be avoided.

CEREALS AND DERIVED PRODUCTS: These are usually foods that you consume daily without even realizing that they contain carbohydratcs. This includes, for example, breakfast cereals, bread, pasta, tortillas, pita, and bagels. Quinoa, barley, buckwheat, rice, and their derivatives are equally forbidden.

LEGUMES AND FRUITS: Most legumes and fruits are not allowed for those who follow the ketogenic diet. The compotes and fruit salads are also part of the elements to avoid. With the exception, the berries can sometimes be consumed according to the state of health of each.

DAIRY PRODUCTS: This includes yogurts, soft cheeses, fresh cheeses, low-fat cheeses and soy products. Whether flavored or natural, these are therefore to be avoided.

PASTRY: In addition to containing cereal products, pastries very often contain added sugar. Among those to avoid are muffins, pancakes, donuts, cookies and different kinds of cakes.

SOME SWEET PRODUCTS: Such as candies but also chocolates are to be avoided during a ketogenic diet. It is also advisable to avoid consuming soft drinks, various sauces containing sugars, as well as cereal coffee.

The ketogenic diet is not just about preventing the foods we love; it's one of the most versatile we have ever seen.

Many tasty recipes and very healthy foods are to put forward for a ketogenic diet. This includes for example:

DAIRY PRODUCTS: This concern, for example, milk that is preferred when it is whole at 3.25%. There are also yogurts which are more recommended if they are natural and with only 7 or 8% of fat.

VEGETABLES: Since carbohydrates are not very much appreciated in this diet, it is better not to pay attention to those who are too much. Among those that are really to be banned are carrots, beets, corn, parsnips, potatoes, sweet potatoes, squash or green peas.

OTHER FOODS TOLERATED: This concerns, for example, wine, alcohol as well as coffee without sugar. As they often contain a large number of carbohydrates, their consumption should be done in small quantities.

Although lipids are an integral part of the ketogenic diet, it is best to pay attention to some of them. Some of the most important are those that contain a high amount of omega-6. These are mainly soybean, corn, safflower, and wheat germ oils.

THE BENEFITS OF THE KETOGENIC DIET

The ketogenic diet has a lot of benefits for our body. Very low in carbohydrate, it is recommended in therapeutic mode against cancer, some forms of epilepsy in children and potentially Alzheimer's disease, Parkinson's, stroke and weight loss, of course. The recommendation is not to consume more than 2g of carbohydrates per 100 gr of food per day. Thus, we replace the 50% carbohydrate of our daily diet with 90% lipid. Green vegetables, fresh fish, and meat are to be favored, as well as unfermented dairy products. Despite the weight loss provided by the ketogenic diet, the muscle mass is not diminished because it will always have the energy necessary for its vitality.

21 Days Meal Plan

Week 1:

	Breakfast	Mid-Morning	Lunch	Dinner	Dessert
Day 1	Breakfast Ketogenic Pancake Muffins	Crispy Chipotle Chicken Thighs	Creamy Meatballs	Ketogenic Mushroom Cauliflower Risotto	Coconut Cake
Day 2	Ketogenic Style Cauliflower Waffles	Keto Tortilla Chips	Quick Cheesy Beef	Creamy Zucchini and Chicken Curry	Ketogenic Style Strawberry Coconut pudding
Day 3	Peanut Butter Breakfast Shake	Coconut Cream Yogurt	Ketogenic Beef Veggie Curry	Beef Casserole	Ketogenic Almond Date Cream Pies
Day 4	Breakfast Ketogenic Pancake Muffins	Ketogenic Sausage Almond Corndogs	Herby Mushroom with Chicken Tenders	Cheesy Leftover pie	Ketogenic Style Lemon Custard
Day 5	Pumpkin Spiced Banana Breakfast Toast	Crispy Chipotle Chicken Thighs	Creamy Meatballs	Ketogenic Mushroom Cauliflower Risotto	Brownies without Flour
Day 6	Breakfast Chicken Sausage with Creamy Scrambled Eggs	Keto Tortilla Chips	Quick Coconut Flavored Pork Chops	Mushroom and Vegetable Curry	Coconut Cake
Day 7	Breakfast Ketogenic Pancake Muffins	Ketogenic Chocolate Almond Cookies	Quick Cheesy Beef	Herby Chicken	Ketogenic Coconut Coffee Ice Cream

Week 2:

	Breakfast	Mid-Morning	Lunch	Dinner	Dessert
Day 8	Breakfast Ketogenic Pancake Muffins	Crispy Chipotle Chicken Thighs	Creamy Meatballs	Cheesy Leftover pie	Ketogenic Style Strawberry Coconut pudding
Day 9	Ketogenic Style Cauliflower Waffles	Ketogenic Sausage Almond Corndogs	Ketogenic Beef Veggie Curry	Beef Casserole	Coconut Cake
Day 10	Pumpkin Spiced Banana Breakfast Toast	Keto Tortilla Chips	Herby Mushroom with Chicken Tenders	Mushroom and Vegetable Curry	Ketogenic Almond Date Cream Pies
Day 11	Breakfast Ketogenic Pancake Muffins	Coconut Cream Yogurt	Creamy Meatballs	Herby Chicken	Brownies without Flour
Day 12	Peanut Butter Breakfast Shake	Crispy Chipotle Chicken Thighs	Quick Cheesy Beef	Ketogenic Mushroom Cauliflower Risotto	Ketogenic Style Lemon Custard
Day 13	Breakfast Chicken Sausage with Creamy Scrambled Eggs	Keto Tortilla Chips	Ketogenic Beef Veggie Curry	Cheesy Leftover pie	Coconut Cake
Day 14	Ketogenic Style Cauliflower Waffles	Ketogenic Sausage Almond Corndogs	Creamy Meatballs	Ketogenic Mushroom Cauliflower Risotto	Ketogenic Coconut Coffee Ice Cream

Week 3:

	Breakfast	Mid-Morning	Lunch	Dinner	Dessert
Day 15	Pumpkin Spiced Banana Breakfast Toast	Crispy Chipotle Chicken Thighs	Quick Cheesy Beef	Creamy Zucchini and Chicken Curry	Ketogenic Style Strawberry Coconut pudding
Day 16	Breakfast Ketogenic Pancake Muffins	Ketogenic Chocolate Almond Cookies	Ketogenic Beef Veggie Curry	Ketogenic Mushroom Cauliflower Risotto	Ketogenic Almond Date Cream Pies
Day 17	Pumpkin Spiced Banana Breakfast Toast	Crispy Chipotle Chicken Thighs	Creamy Meatballs	Mushroom and Vegetable Curry	Coconut Cake
Day 18	Ketogenic Style Cauliflower Waffles	Coconut Cream Yogurt	Quick Coconut Flavored Pork Chops	Creamy Zucchini and Chicken Curry	Ketogenic Style Lemon Custard
Day 19	Peanut Butter Breakfast Shake	Ketogenic Chocolate Almond Cookies	Herby Mushroom with Chicken Tenders	Ketogenic Mushroom Cauliflower Risotto	Brownies without Flour
Day 20	Breakfast Ketogenic Pancake Muffins	Keto Tortilla Chips	Creamy Meatballs	Mushroom and Vegetable Curry	Coconut Cake
Day 21	Pumpkin Spiced Banana Breakfast Toast	Coconut Cream Yogurt	Quick Cheesy Beef	Cheesy Leftover pie	Ketogenic Almond Date Cream Pies

Ketogenic Recipes

Breakfast

Breakfast Ketogenic Pancake Muffins

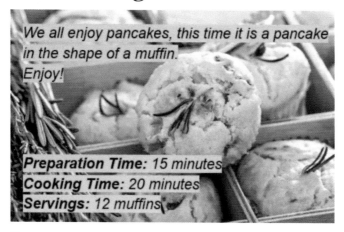

We all enjoy pancakes, this time it is a pancake in the shape of a muffin. Enjoy!

Preparation Time: 15 minutes
Cooking Time: 20 minutes
Servings: 12 muffins

Ingredients:

6 ounces ground sausage

4 tablespoons maple syrup

1½ cup almond flour

1 teaspoon vanilla extract

¼ teaspoon salt

1 teaspoon baking powder

4 tablespoons coconut milk

2 tablespoons psyllium husk powder

20 drops liquid Stevia

4 eggs

¼ cup erythritol

Directions:

1. Preheat your oven to 350 degrees F.
2. Cut the sausage into thin circles.
3. In a pan sear the sausage slightly.
4. In a mixing bowl, combine all the dry ingredients.
5. In another bowl, combine all the wet ingredients.
6. Add the wet ingredients with the dry ingredients and mix well.
7. Add the seared sausage and mix well.
8. Pour the mixture into muffin cups.
9. Bake in the preheated oven for about 20 minutes.
10. Serve warm.

Nutrition Facts: (per serving)

160.5 Calories/ 12.88g Fats/ 2.16g Net Carbs/ 7.6g Protein

Peanut Butter Breakfast Shake

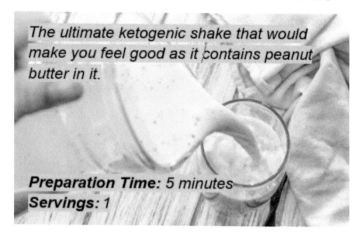

The ultimate ketogenic shake that would make you feel good as it contains peanut butter in it.

Preparation Time: 5 minutes
Servings: 1

Ingredients:

1 cup Coconut Milk

2 tablespoon salted caramel

7 ice Cubes

1 tablespoon coconut oil

2 tablespoon Peanut Butter

4 teaspoon Xanthan gum

Directions:

1. In a blender add the coconut milk, peanut butter.
2. Add the salted caramel, coconut oil, and xanthan gum.
3. Blend for about 30 seconds and add the ice cubes.
4. Blend for another minute.
5. Serve fresh.

Nutrition Facts: (per serving)

369 Calories/ 34.95g Fats/ 7.53g Net Carbs/ 8.1g Protein

Ketogenic Style Cauliflower Waffles

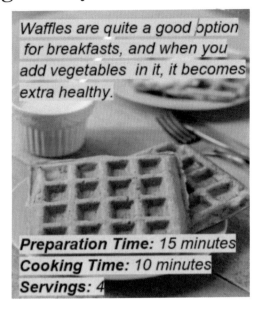

Waffles are quite a good option for breakfasts, and when you add vegetables in it, it becomes extra healthy.

Preparation Time: 15 minutes
Cooking Time: 10 minutes
Servings: 4

Ingredients:

½ large head cauliflower

2 eggs

1 cup packed collard greens

2 stalks green onion

1/3 cup Parmesan cheese

1 tablespoon sesame seed

1 tablespoon olive oil

½ teaspoon ground black pepper

2 teaspoons fresh chopped thyme

1 cup finely shredded mozzarella cheese

1 teaspoon garlic powder

½ teaspoon salt

Directions:

1. In a blender add the cauliflower and blend until it becomes grainy.

2. Add the spring onion, collard greens, thyme and blend for another minute.

3. Transfer the mix into a mixing bowl.

4. Add the remaining ingredients.

5. Mix well and make your waffles using a waffle maker.

6. Serve hot.

Nutrition Facts: *(per serving)*

203.25 Calories/ 15.38g Fats/ 5.86g Net Carbs/ 14.99g Protein

Breakfast Chicken Sausage with Creamy Scrambled Eggs

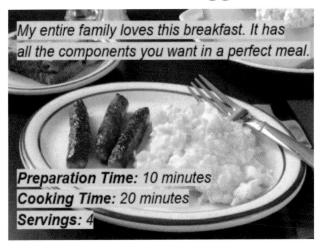

My entire family loves this breakfast. It has all the components you want in a perfect meal.

Preparation Time: 10 minutes
Cooking Time: 20 minutes
Servings: 4

Ingredients:

4 slices chicken sausage

3 eggs

1 tablespoon butter

Pinch of salt

1/3 cup heavy whipping cream

Pinch of freshly ground black pepper

Directions:

1. Preheat your oven to 350 degrees F.
2. Arrange the chicken sausage on a baking sheet.
3. Bake 10 minutes or until crispy.
4. Whisk the eggs in a bowl.

5. Add the cream and whisk lightly.

6. In a saucepan add a little oil and melt on low heat.

7. Add the egg mixture and allow it to cook for 2 minutes.

8. Mix with a spatula and cook for another minute.

9. Serve eggs with chicken sausage.

Nutrition Facts: *(per serving)*

761 Calories/ 68.15g Fats/ 3.68g Net Carbs/ 32.77g Protein

Goat Cheese and Leftover Salmon Breakfast Delight

Goat cheese is very good for health, so is salmon. Combine these two, and you get a super breakfast.

Preparation Time: 15 minutes
Servings: 4

Ingredients:

4 ounces smoked salmon

1 cup goat cheese, softened

½ cup Arugula.

½ cup of shredded Radicchio

1-2 cloves garlic

1 tablespoon fresh rosemary

1 tablespoon fresh basil

Salt, pepper and avocado oil to taste

Directions:

1. In a bowl, combine the goat cheese with garlic, herbs, salt, and pepper.

2. Mix well and set aside for now.

3. Rinse the Radicchio and the Arugula.

4. Add smoked salmon and goat cheese mixture on top.

5. Black pepper and avocado oil for serving.

Nutrition Facts: *(per serving)*

46.19 Calories/ 3.33g Fats/ 0.94g Net Carbs/ 3.43g Protein

Pumpkin Spiced Banana Breakfast Toast

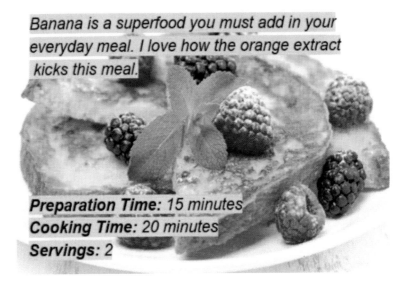

Banana is a superfood you must add in your everyday meal. I love how the orange extract kicks this meal.

Preparation Time: 15 minutes
Cooking Time: 20 minutes
Servings: 2

Ingredients:

4 slices Banana bread

¼ teaspoon pumpkin pie spice

1 egg

1/8 teaspoon orange extract

½ teaspoon vanilla extract

2 tablespoons cream

2 tablespoons butter

Directions:

1. In a bowl, whisk the egg.

2. Add the pumpkin pie spice, orange extract, and vanilla extract.

3. Mix well, add the cream, and mix again.

4. Dip each bread slice in the egg mixture.

5. In a pan melt the butter and fry the banana bread slices golden brown from both sides.

Nutrition Facts: *(per 2 slice)*

429.73 Calories/ 36.7g Fats/ 7.33g Net Carbs/ 13.36g Protein

Lunch

Chicken Thighs with Creamy Veggies

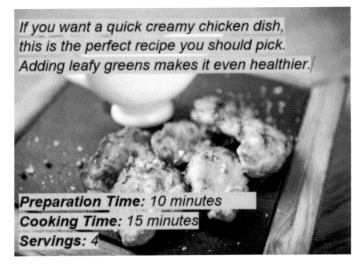

If you want a quick creamy chicken dish, this is the perfect recipe you should pick. Adding leafy greens makes it even healthier.

Preparation Time: 10 minutes
Cooking Time: 15 minutes
Servings: 4

Ingredients:

1 lb chicken thighs

1 teaspoon Italian herbs

2 Tablespoon coconut oil

1 cup cream

2 cups spinach / arugula or other dark leafy greens

Salt and pepper, to taste

2 Tablespoon butter, melted

1 cup chicken stock

2 Tablespoon coconut flour

Directions:

1. Discard the bones of the chicken. Keep the skin. Season with salt and pepper.

2. In a skillet, heat some coconut oil.

3. Sear the chicken thighs until browned. Arrange on serving plate.

4. To make the sauce, melt the butter in a pan.

5. Add coconut flour and stir continuously.

6. Add cream and bring it to a boil.

7. Add the herbs and pour in the chicken stock.

8. Add the greens and stir for 2 minutes.

9. Remove heat and serve with chicken.

Nutrition Facts: *(per serving)*

446 Calories/ 38.19g Fats/ 2.61g Net Carbs/ 18.42g Protein

Creamy Meatballs

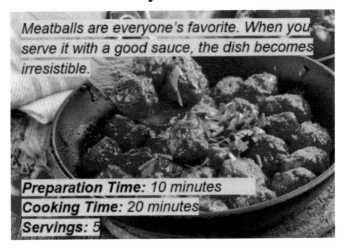

Meatballs are everyone's favorite. When you serve it with a good sauce, the dish becomes irresistible.

Preparation Time: 10 minutes
Cooking Time: 20 minutes
Servings: 5

Ingredients:

The meatballs

1 pound ground beef

¼ cup Parmesan cheese

1 egg

½ teaspoon onion powder

For the sauce

1/3 cup sugar-free ketchup

1 ½ cups water

1 cup erythritol

¼ cup apple cider vinegar

3 tablespoons soy sauce

½ teaspoon xanthan gum

Directions:

1. Combine the beef, onion, cheese, and egg in a bowl.
2. Mix well and create meatballs using your hands.
3. In a pan, brown the meatballs over medium-low heat.
4. Transfer them onto a plate.
5. Using the same pan, combine apple cider vinegar, water, soy sauce, erythritol, and sugar-free ketchup.
6. Mix well until the sauce thickens.
7. Add the xanthan gum slowly and mix well.
8. Simmer for 5 minutes and add the meatballs.

Cook for additional 5 minutes and serve hot.

Nutrition Facts: *(per serving)*

295.4 Calories/ 18.66g Fats/ 5.35g Net Carbs/ 28.26g Protein

Quick Cheesy Beef

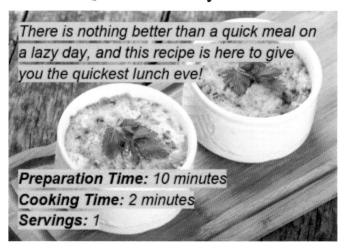

There is nothing better than a quick meal on a lazy day, and this recipe is here to give you the quickest lunch eve!

Preparation Time: 10 minutes
Cooking Time: 2 minutes
Servings: 1

Ingredients:

1.5 ounces pepper jack cheese, shredded

1.5 tablespoons diced green chiles

2 ounces roast beef deli slices

1 tablespoon sour cream

Directions:

1. Arrange 1/3 of the beef slices onto your mug.
2. Add half of the sour cream.
3. Add half of the green chiles.
4. Add 1/3 of the cheese.
5. Now repeat with another layer of everything. The top should have cheese.
6. Add to your microwave.

7. Microwave for only 2 minutes.

8. Serve hot.

Nutrition Facts: *(per serving)*

268 Calories/ 17.99g Fats/ 3.83g Net Carbs/ 22.4g Protein

Ketogenic Beef Veggie Curry

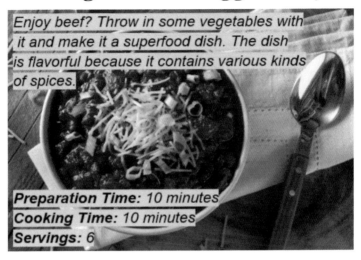

Enjoy beef? Throw in some vegetables with it and make it a superfood dish. The dish is flavorful because it contains various kinds of spices.

Preparation Time: 10 minutes
Cooking Time: 10 minutes
Servings: 6

Ingredients:

2 lbs. Ground Beef

1/4 cup Parmesan Cheese

8 cups Spinach

2/3 onion, chopped

1 Tablespoon Olive Oil

1 cup tomato sauce

2 teaspoon Cayenne Pepper

2 Green Bell Peppers, diced

1 1/2 Tablespoon Chili Powder

1 teaspoon Garlic Powder

1 Tablespoon Cumin

Salt and Pepper to Taste

Directions:

1. In a pressure cooker add the onion with oil and toss for a few seconds.

2. Add the bell peppers and toss for few more seconds.

3. Season using salt and pepper. Transfer to a plate.

4. Add the beef and stir until browned.

5. Season using all the spice and salt.

6. Finally add the stirred vegetables, spinach, tomato sauce and mix well.

7. Cover and cook on low heat for 5 minutes.

8. Add the cheese and let it melt.

9. Serve warm.

Nutrition Facts: *(per serving)*

404.33 Calories/ 27.06g Fat/ 5.11g Carbs/ 31.09g Protein

Quick Coconut Flavored Pork Chops

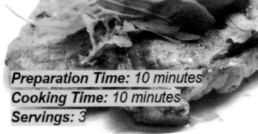

Add some fun to your regular pork chop recipe by adding coconut flavor in it. Not at all complicated, and you can dish out this recipe within 20 minutes.

Preparation Time: 10 minutes
Cooking Time: 10 minutes
Servings: 3

Ingredients:

Crust

1 1/2 lb. Pork Chops

1 teaspoon Coriander

2 tablespoon shredded coconut

2 teaspoon Cumin

1 teaspoon Cardamom

3 Tablespoon Coconut Oil

1/4 Cup Golden Flaxseed

Salt, Pepper

Vegetables

1/4 Cup White Wine

1 Orange Pepper

Salt, Pepper

1/2 Onion

2 Stalks Celery

Directions:

1. Use salt and pepper to season the pork chops.

2. In a bowl add all the crust ingredients. Mix well.

3. Add the pork chops into the crust mixture. Let it sit for 10 minutes.

4. In a cast iron skillet cook the pork chops until they are nice and crispy.

5. In a pot add the orange pepper, onion, celery, white wine, and seasoning.

6. Cook for 5 minutes and serve with the pork chops.

Nutrition Facts: (per serving)

439 Calories/ 23.7g Fats/ 4.3g Net Carbs/ 50.3g Protein

Herby Mushroom with Chicken Tenders

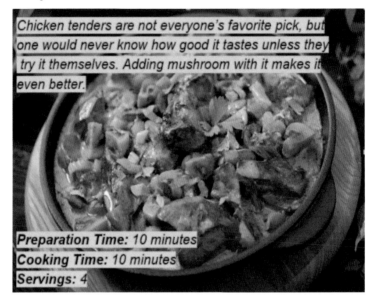

Chicken tenders are not everyone's favorite pick, but one would never know how good it tastes unless they try it themselves. Adding mushroom with it makes it even better.

Preparation Time: 10 minutes
Cooking Time: 10 minutes
Servings: 4

Ingredients:

1 cup white button mushrooms, diced

1 cup chicken broth

3 cloves garlic

1 pound chicken tenders, cubed

½ teaspoon dried basil

Salt and pepper to taste

½ teaspoon dried oregano

¼ cup chopped fresh parsley

¼ teaspoon dried thyme

2 bay leaves

¼ cup heavy whipping cream

2 tablespoons butter

Directions:

1. In a pressure cooker add the mushrooms.
2. Add the chicken tenders, all the herbs, broth, salt, pepper, garlic and cover.
3. Cook for only 10 minutes.
4. Add butter, cream and mix well.
5. Take off the heat and serve with herbs on top.

Nutrition Facts: *(per serving)*

297.2 Calories/ 17.5g Fats/ 4.42g Net Carbs/ 29.99g Protein

Dinner

Ketogenic Mushroom Cauliflower Risotto

Risotto is one such dish, no matter which part of the earth you are in, you would love it and probably ate it at one point. Risotto is famous in a different nation with different names.

Preparation Time: 10 minutes
Cooking Time: 10 minutes
Servings: 4

Ingredients:

1 cup finely chopped cauliflower (stem removed)

½ cup chicken broth

3 mushrooms, sliced

½ teaspoon garlic powder

¼ cup sliced almonds

¼ teaspoon dried parsley

2 tablespoons butter

Salt and pepper to taste

Directions:

1. In a pan melt the butter and fry the mushrooms for 20 seconds.

2. Add the almonds, cauliflower, broth, salt, and pepper.

3. Stir well and add the parsley.

4. Stir for about 8 minutes.

5. Serve hot.

Nutrition Facts: *(per serving)*

311.5 Calories/ 28.25g Fats/ 3.11g Net Carbs/ 15.4g Protein

Cheesy Leftover pie

Whenever I have leftover meat, I always think of pies. This is like the ultimate comfort food for my family and me.

Preparation Time: 10 minutes
Cooking Time: 12 minutes
Servings: 4

Ingredients:

½ cup leftover meat

1 ¼ cups mozzarella cheese

4 tablespoons almond flour

3 tablespoons coconut flour

3.5 ounces cheddar cheese

1 egg

1 teaspoon Italian seasoning

Salt and pepper to taste

Directions:

1. Preheat your oven to 450 degrees F.
2. Shred the mozzarella cheese.
3. Microwave the mozzarella cheese for 30 seconds.
4. In a bowl combine the flours with salt and pepper.
5. Add the melted cheese, egg and mix well.
6. Arrange parchment paper onto a flat surface.
7. Roll out the mixture and create two 6 inch round disk.
8. Add the filling onto one round disk.
9. Top with another round disk and seal the edges carefully.
10. Add to the oven and bake for 10 minutes.
11. Serve warm.

Nutrition Facts: *(per serving)*

322.5 Calories/ 22.23g Fats/ 4.98g Net Carbs/ 22.67g Protein

Mushroom and Vegetable Curry

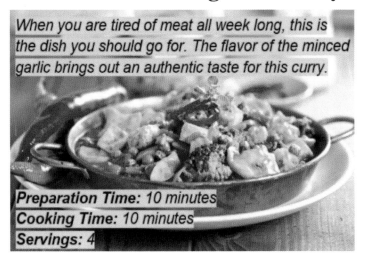

When you are tired of meat all week long, this is the dish you should go for. The flavor of the minced garlic brings out an authentic taste for this curry.

Preparation Time: 10 minutes
Cooking Time: 10 minutes
Servings: 4

Ingredients:

1 cup mushrooms

2 teaspoons minced garlic

115g broccoli

90g bell pepper

6 tablespoons olive oil

2 tablespoons pumpkin seeds

1 teaspoon salt

100g sugar snap peas

90g spinach

½ teaspoon red pepper flakes

1 teaspoon pepper

Directions:

1. Cut all the vegetables in the same size.
2. In a pressure cooker add the oil and fry the garlic.
3. Add the mushrooms (can be substituted with Tofu) and vegetables
4. Add the remaining ingredients.
5. Cover and cook for 8 minutes.
6. Serve hot.

Nutrition Facts: *(per serving)*

235.5 Calories/ 21.2g Fats/ 6.37g Net Carbs/ 4.26g Protein

Herby Chicken

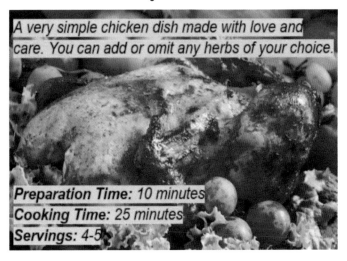

A very simple chicken dish made with love and care. You can add or omit any herbs of your choice.

Preparation Time: 10 minutes
Cooking Time: 25 minutes
Servings: 4-5

Ingredients

5 pound chicken

4 tablespoons butter, softened

Salt and pepper to taste

1 whole lemon

1 tablespoon dried parsley

1 small bunch fresh thyme

1 small bunch fresh oregano

1 tablespoon olive oil

Directions

1. Preheat your oven to 450 degrees F.

2. Use a kitchen towel to pat chicken dry.

3. Season the chicken's inside using oregano, salt, thyme, and pepper.

4. Add lemon inside. Tie the legs together using a thread.

5. Brush half of the melted butter onto the skin and season using salt and pepper.

6. Add to the oven and roast for 15 minutes.

7. Reduce the temperature to 325 degrees F and bake for another 10 minutes.

8. Do not waste any juice that may come out, brush it generously onto the bird.

9. Add parsley and serve warm.

Nutrition Facts: *(per serving)*

429.88 Calories/ 30.45g Fats/ 5.1g Net Carbs/ 32.95g Protein

Beef Casserole

A classic casserole dish, which is ketogenic friendly. You can substitute the beef with mutton or chicken. You can also make it vegetarian if you wish.

Preparation Time: 10 minutes
Cooking Time: 25 minutes
Servings: 4

Ingredients:

1 lb. Ground Beef

1 cup Cheddar Cheese

265g Cauliflower

1/2 teaspoon Garlic Powder

1 tablespoon Dijon Mustard

1/2 teaspoon Onion Powder

2 tablespoon tomato puree

Salt and Pepper to Taste

2 tablespoon Mayonnaise

1/2 cup almond flour

3 eggs

Directions:

1. Preheat the oven to 350 degrees F.

2. In a blender add the cauliflower and blend until grainy.

3. Add the beef and make it crumbly.

4. In a pan add the mixture and cook for 5 minutes.

5. In a bowl, transfer the mixture.

6. Add all the ingredients excluding the cheese.

7. Add the mixture onto your baking dish.

8. Top using the cheese.

9. Bake in the oven for 20 minutes.

10. Serve warm.

Nutrition Facts: *(per serving)*

478 Calories/ 35.5g Fats/ 3.6g Net Carbs/ 32.2g Protein

Creamy Zucchini and Chicken Curry

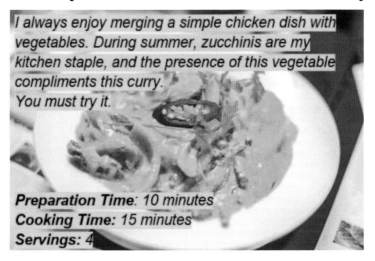

I always enjoy merging a simple chicken dish with vegetables. During summer, zucchinis are my kitchen staple, and the presence of this vegetable compliments this curry.
You must try it.

Preparation Time: 10 minutes
Cooking Time: 15 minutes
Servings: 4

Ingredients:

4 ounces softened cream cheese

2 pound chicken, shredded

2 ¼ cups pepper jack cheese

1 yellow bell pepper, diced

¼ white onion, diced

1 red bell pepper, diced

2 teaspoons olive oil

1 teaspoon garlic powder

3 medium zucchini, spiralizer

1 cup heavy cream

¼ cup water

Salt and pepper to taste

Directions:

1. In a pressure cooker add the oil and fry the onion for 2 minutes.

2. Add the chicken and toss for another minute.

3. Add the garlic powder, salt, pepper, and water.

4. Stir well and cover with lid.

5. Cook for 5 minutes and add the heavy cream, cream cheese, and jack cheese.

6. Cook for another 5 minutes and serve.

Nutrition Facts: *(per serving)*

554 Calories/ 40.17g Fats/ 6.37g Net Carbs/ 34.15g Protein

Snack

Egg Stuffed Portobello Mushrooms

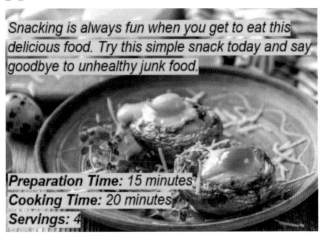

Snacking is always fun when you get to eat this delicious food. Try this simple snack today and say goodbye to unhealthy junk food.

Preparation Time: 15 minutes
Cooking Time: 20 minutes
Servings: 4

Ingredients:

4 large Portobello mushrooms

Salt and pepper to taste

2 ounces cream cheese

2 eggs

1/3 cup shredded Parmesan cheese

2.5 tablespoons olive oil

5 Cups spinach

2 tablespoons flax seed meal

Directions:

1. Preheat the oven to 400 degrees F.

2. Cut the stem off the mushrooms and scoop out the flesh.

3. Arrange them on a sheet pan.

4. Brush olive oil on top of the mushroom caps.

5. Sprinkle some salt and pepper.

6. Bake the mushrooms for about 10 minutes.

7. Hard boil the eggs and let them cool down.

8. Discard the shell and chop them finely.

9. In a pan toss the spinach for just 1 minute and add the cream cheese.

10. Add half of the parmesan cheese and season using salt and pepper.

11. Take off the heat and add the chopped eggs.

12. Stuff the mushrooms using the cheese filling.

13. Add flax seed meal and cheese on top of each mushroom.

14. Bake for about 5 minutes.

15. Serve warm.

Nutrition Facts: *(per serving)*

245.25 Calories/ 21.41g Fats/ 3.36g Net Carbs/ 10.81g Protein

Ketogenic Sausage Almond Corndogs

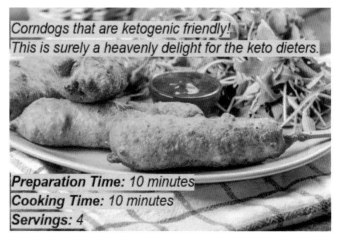

Corndogs that are ketogenic friendly!
This is surely a heavenly delight for the keto dieters.

Preparation Time: 10 minutes
Cooking Time: 10 minutes
Servings: 4

Ingredients:

1 Cup almond meal

1/2 teaspoon turmeric

2 tablespoon heavy cream

2 eggs

4 sausages

1 teaspoon baking powder

1/2 teaspoon salt

1 1/2 cups olive oil

1/4 teaspoon cayenne pepper

Directions:

1. In a bowl, combine the spices with the almond meal and baking powder.

2. In another bowl, whisk the eggs.

3. Add the heavy cream to it.

4. Combine the egg mix with the almond meal mix.

5. In a skillet, heat the olive oil over medium-high heat.

6. Take each sausage and dip into the almond mixture.

7. Fry them golden brown. It may take about 2 minutes per side.

8. Serve hot with any sauce of your choice.

Nutrition Facts: *(per serving)*

493.75 Calories/ 45.93g Fats/ 4.52g Net Carbs/ 15.4g Protein

Ketogenic Chocolate Almond Cookie

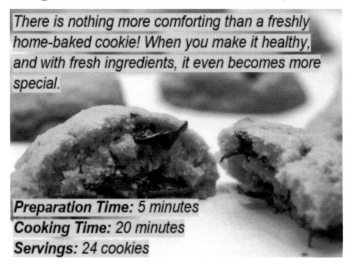

There is nothing more comforting than a freshly home-baked cookie! When you make it healthy, and with fresh ingredients, it even becomes more special.

Preparation Time: 5 minutes
Cooking Time: 20 minutes
Servings: 24 cookies

Ingredients:

½ cup almond flakes

2 tablespoons Scotch

½ cup erythritol

1 egg

½ cup softened butter

1 teaspoon baking powder

1½ cup almond flour

3.5 ounces unsweetened bakers chocolate

½ teaspoon vanilla extract

Directions:

1. In a large mixing bowl, combine the almond flour, baking powder.

2. In another bowl beat the egg.

3. Add the vanilla, scotch, erythritol, butter, and mix until it becomes creamy.

4. Combine the egg mix with the flour mix.

5. Add the chopped chocolate and almond flakes.

6. Fold gently and knead into dough.

7. Add to the fridge for 20 minutes.

8. Roll them onto a flat surface and cut into cookie shapes.

9. Preheat the oven to 325 degrees F.

10. Arrange the cookies onto a baking sheet.

11. Bake for about 20 minutes.

12. Serve in room temperature.

Nutrition Facts: (per serving)

117.24 Calories/ 10.62g Fats/ 1.36g Net Carbs/ 3.13g Protein

Keto Tortilla Chips

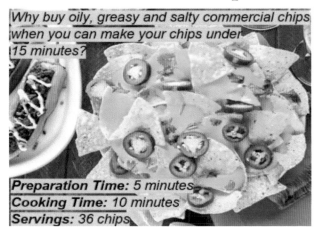

Why buy oily, greasy and salty commercial chips when you can make your chips under 15 minutes?

Preparation Time: 5 minutes
Cooking Time: 10 minutes
Servings: 36 chips

Ingredients:

6 readymade tortillas

Salt and pepper to taste

Oil for deep-frying

Directions:

1. Use a pizza cutter to cut the tortillas into slices.
2. Preheat the deep fryer.
3. Fry the tortillas into batches for 2 minutes per side.
4. Transfer to a kitchen towel.
5. Sprinkle some salt, pepper or any other spice blend of your choice on top.

Nutrition Facts: *(per serving)*

40.34 Calories/ 3.03g Fats/ 0.37g Net Carbs/ 0.83g Protein.

Coconut Cream Yogurt

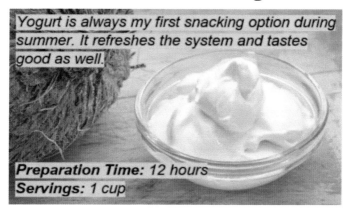

Yogurt is always my first snacking option during summer. It refreshes the system and tastes good as well.

Preparation Time: 12 hours
Servings: 1 cup

Ingredients:

1 can coconut milk

½ teaspoon Xanthan Gum

2/3 cup heavy whipping cream

Directions:

1. In a mixing bowl, combine the coconut milk with whipping cream.
2. Mix well and add the xanthan gum.
3. Mix well and add to an ovenproof dish.
4. Preheat the oven for 10 minutes over 400 degrees F.
5. Cover the top using a lid and add the dish to the oven.
6. Turn off the oven and let the yogurt set for 12 hours.
7. Let it cool down in the refrigerator for 2 hours.

Nutrition Facts*: per 1/2 cup*

314.75 Calories/ 32.17g Fats/ 4.08g Net Carbs/ 1.16g Protein

Crispy Chipotle Chicken Thighs

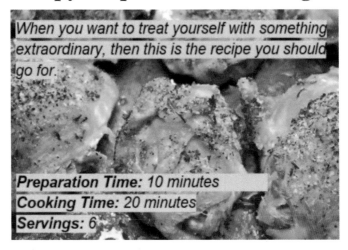

When you want to treat yourself with something extraordinary, then this is the recipe you should go for.

Preparation Time: 10 minutes
Cooking Time: 20 minutes
Servings: 6

Ingredients

6 chicken thighs

1/2 teaspoon chipotle powder

1/2 teaspoon onion powder

1/4 teaspoon cumin

1/2 teaspoon coriander

1/2 teaspoon smoked paprika

1/2 teaspoon garlic powder

Pinch cayenne

1 tablespoon olive oil

Salt and pepper to taste

1/4 teaspoon oregano

Directions

1. In a bowl, combine all the spices.

2. Discard the bones of the chicken thighs.

3. Season the chicken using oil, salt, pepper and the spice mixture.

4. Add some oil onto a skillet and heat over a medium high flame.

5. Add the chicken pieces with their skin side down.

6. Cook for 10 minutes and then flip.

7. Cook for another 5 minutes and take off the heat and serve with any sauce.

Nutrition Facts: *(per serving)*

597 Calories/ 53.5g Fats/ 1g Net Carb/ 28g Protein

Bonus Dessert

Coconut Cake

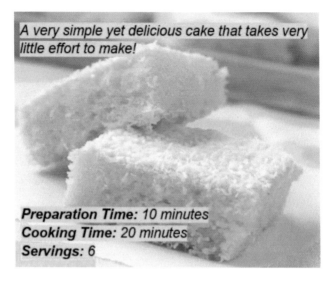

A very simple yet delicious cake that takes very little effort to make!

Preparation Time: 10 minutes
Cooking Time: 20 minutes
Servings: 6

Ingredients:

8 Eggs

2/3 cup Whole Grain Soy Flour

1/4 teaspoon Salt

1 teaspoon Baking Powder

1 cup butter

2/3 cup Dried Coconut

1 1/2 cups Sucralose

3 teaspoon Coconut Extract

Directions:

1. Heat oven to 350 degrees F.

2. Use cooking spray to grease your cake pan.

3. Melt the butter and set aside for now.

4. Beat the eggs with sugar.

5. Add coconut extracts and whip until starts to thicken and you can see ribbons forming in it.

6. Add the butter and beat again.

7. Shift the dry ingredients into the mixture and fold gently.

8. Pour into your cake pan and bake for about 20 minutes.

9. Serve in room temperature.

Nutrition Facts: *(per serving)*

397 Calories/ 38g Fats/ 5.8g Net Carb/ 8g Protein

Brownies without Flour

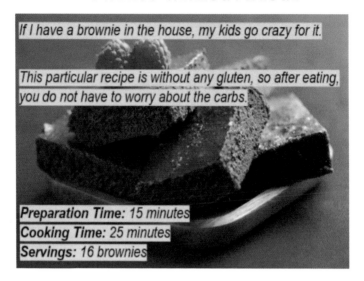

If I have a brownie in the house, my kids go crazy for it.

This particular recipe is without any gluten, so after eating, you do not have to worry about the carbs.

Preparation Time: 15 minutes
Cooking Time: 25 minutes
Servings: 16 brownies

Ingredients:

5 ounces low-carb milk chocolate

¼ cup mascarpone cheese

3 eggs

¼ cup unsweetened cocoa powder

4 tablespoons butter

½ teaspoon salt

½ cup Swerve

Directions:

1. Preheat your oven to 375 degrees F.
2. Arrange parchment paper onto your baking pan.
3. Melt the chocolate in a double boiler.
4. Melt the butter and let it cool down.
5. Whish the eggs with the swerve and make a frothy mixture.
6. Add the cheese and beat well.
7. Add the salt and half of the cocoa powder.
8. Add the melted chocolate and mix well.
9. Add to your baking pan.
10. Bake for about 25 minutes. Serve in room temperature.

Nutrition Facts: *(per serving)*

86.94 Calories/ 8.05g Fat/ 2.9g Net Carbs/ 2.18g Protein

Ketogenic Style Lemon Custard

This is definitely a luxurious custard according to me. I relish it when I want to give my tummy a treat.

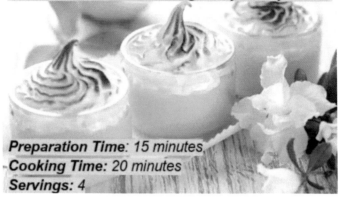

Preparation Time: 15 minutes
Cooking Time: 20 minutes
Servings: 4

Ingredients:

For the Custard

1/3 cup stevia - erythritol blend

1 ½ cups heavy whipping cream

½ teaspoon xanthan gum

½ teaspoon vanilla extract

Pinch of salt

Zest from 2 lemons

½ teaspoon lemon extract

2 egg yolks

For the Meringue

1 tablespoon stevia - erythritol blend

2 egg whites

1/8 teaspoon vanilla extract

1/8 teaspoon cream of tartar

Directions:

1. In a pan, combine the xanthan gum, lemon zest, salt and 1/3 cup of sweetener.
2. Heat over medium-low heat and mix well.
3. Add the heavy cream and switch to low heat.
4. Add the egg yolks and keep stirring.
5. Add the lemon extract and vanilla extract.
6. Mix well and pour the mix into your ramekins.
7. To make the meringue, beat the egg whites.
8. Add the cream of tartar and beat until it forms soft peaks.
9. Add the remaining sweetener, and beat again.
10. Add on top of the custard and broil in the oven for about 20 seconds.
11. Serve cold.

Nutrition Facts: *(per serving)*

353.87 Calories/ 35.38g Fats/ 2.85g Net Carbs/ 4.97g Protein

Ketogenic Coconut Coffee Ice Cream

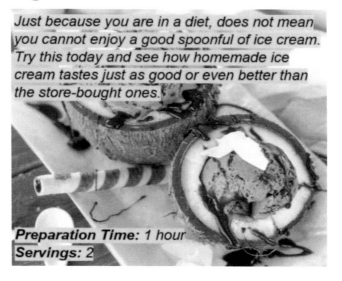

Just because you are in a diet, does not mean you cannot enjoy a good spoonful of ice cream. Try this today and see how homemade ice cream tastes just as good or even better than the store-bought ones.

Preparation Time: 1 hour
Servings: 2

Ingredients:

1 tablespoon Instant Coffee

1/4 cup Heavy Cream

15 drops Liquid Stevia

2 tablespoon Erythritol

1 cup Coconut Milk

2 tablespoon Cocoa Powder

1/4 teaspoon Xanthan Gum

Directions:

1. In a blender, add the instant coffee, cocoa powder, stevia, erythritol, heavy cream and coconut milk.

2. Blend for 2 minutes.

3. Add the xanthan gum and blend until the mixture is slightly thick.

4. Transfer the mixture to your ice cream machine.

5. Follow the icemaker's instruction.

6. Serve the ice cream cold.

Nutrition Facts: *(per serving)*

175 Calories/ 14.98g Fats/ 6.62g Net Carbs/ 2.59g Protein

Ketogenic Style Strawberry Coconut pudding

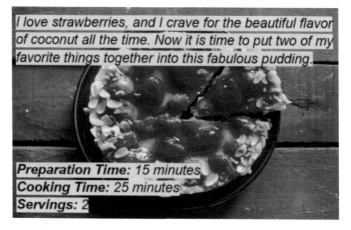

I love strawberries, and I crave for the beautiful flavor of coconut all the time. Now it is time to put two of my favorite things together into this fabulous pudding.

Preparation Time: 15 minutes
Cooking Time: 25 minutes
Servings: 2

Ingredients:

1/4 cup Coconut Flour

1/4 cup strawberries

5 egg Yolks

2 teaspoon Lemon Juice

2 tablespoon Coconut Oil

Zest 1 Lemon

1/4 teaspoon Baking Powder

2 tablespoon erythritol

2 tablespoon Butter

2 tablespoon Heavy Cream

10 drops Liquid Stevia

Directions:

1. Preheat your oven to 350 degrees F.
2. Combine the dry ingredients in a bowl and set aside for now.
3. Divide the egg yolks from egg whites.
4. In a bowl beat the yolks until pale.
5. Add stevia, erythritol and beat again.
6. Add lemon juice, coconut oil, lemon zest, butter and heavy cream.
7. Beat well and then slowly add the dry ingredients.
8. Pour the batter into ramekins and add the strawberries.
9. Bake in the oven for about 25 minutes.

Nutrition Facts: (per serving)

459.5 Calories/ 44.04g Fats/ 4.91g Net Carbs/ 9.1g Protein

Ketogenic Almond Date Cream Pies

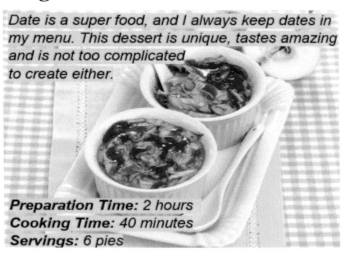

Date is a super food, and I always keep dates in my menu. This dessert is unique, tastes amazing and is not too complicated to create either.

Preparation Time: 2 hours
Cooking Time: 40 minutes
Servings: 6 pies

Ingredients:

The Crust

¼ cup almond flakes

½ cup almond flour

4 tablespoons butter

¼ cup sugar substitute

The Custard

½ cup water

2 egg yolks

1 cup heavy whipping cream

¼ cup almond flour

1 teaspoon vanilla extract

¼ cup sugar substitute

The Top

1 cup heavy whipping cream

1 teaspoon vanilla extract

4 dates, pit removed, chopped

2 tablespoons sugar substitute

Directions:

1. In a pot, melt your butter over low flame.
2. Add the sugar substitute and stir continuously.
3. In a bowl combine, the almond flakes with almond flour and add to the pot.
4. Add 1 tablespoon of the mixture onto each ramekin.
5. Add the cream onto the pot.
6. Add the vanilla and mix.
7. Beat the egg yolks until slurry in a bowl.
8. Add the almond flour and water.
9. Add the egg mixture to the pot and mix well.
10. Take off the heat and let it cool down for 10 minutes.
11. Pour into the ramekins and put in the fridge for 1 hour or 2.
12. For the topping, beat the cream, sugar substitute, vanilla using a beater.
13. Add the dates and beat again.
14. Add the topping and serve.

Nutrition Facts: *(per serving)*

584 Calories/ 57.33g Fats/ 7.25g Net Carbs/ 9.22g Protein

Shopping List

Meat and eggs:
beef
chicken
sausage
pork
eggs

Seafood:
shrimp
salmon

Vegetable:
onion
cauliflowers
collard greens
broccoli
bell pepper
tomatoes
zucchini
chilies
mushroom

Fruits and Nuts:
strawberries

almond

Dairy:
sour cream
packet cream
goat cheese
milk
cream cheese
mozzarella cheese

Vegetable oil:
coconut oil
olive oil
avocado oil

Grocery and other:
brown rice
wheat flour
soy flour
coconut milk
peanut butter
Ketogenic Butter
maple syrup
vanilla extract
coconut extract
ketchup

baking powder
Ketogenic sugar substitute
chocolate chips
liquid Stevia
psyllium husk powder
xanthan Gum
mushroom
readymade Tortilla
Ketogenic Friendly pastry

Herbs:
thyme
rosemary
parsley
italian Herbs
oregano

Spices:
salt
sesame seeds
black pepper
garlic powder.

Printed in Great Britain
by Amazon

79652839R00042